MW00682547

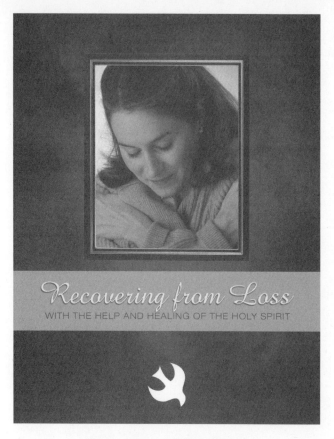

Recovering from Loss
WITH THE HELP AND HEALING OF THE HOLY SPIRIT

SID WATERMAN

HighWay

A division of Anomalos Publishing House

Crane

HighWay

A division of Anomalos Publishing House, Crane 65633

© 2008 by Sid Waterman

All rights reserved. Published 2008

Printed in the United States of America

08 1

ISBN-10: 0981509142 (paper)

EAN-13: 9780981509143 (paper)

Cover illustration and design by Steve Warner

A CIP catalog record for this book is available from the Library of Congress.

About the Author

Sid Waterman is a graduate of the University of Alberta, Edmonton, Canada. In 1970, he received a master of divinity degree from Southern (Baptist Theological) Seminary in Louisville, Kentucky.

For more than thirty years, he pastored churches in western Canada. Since 1994, Sid has been a certified grief recovery counselor in Penticton, B.C., Canada. His work as a grief counselor for Providence Funeral Homes includes making appointments and visiting on a weekly basis those who are suffering a deep loss. This book was not forged in a classroom but in the homes and apartments of those who have suffered broken hearts and vanquished dreams. It is Mr. Waterman's prayer that not only will your mind be enlightened by the truths in this book but that you will also encounter the living God in all His compassion and healing power.

Mr. Waterman has been married to his wife, Pegi, for more than forty years. He has two married sons; Mark and his wife Becky, Chris and wife Stephanie. Their five grandchildren are the delight of their lives.

From 1970–1973, Mr. Phillip Keller, author of *A Shepherd Looks at Psalm 23*, was pastoral assistant to Mr. Waterman. Mr. Keller's deep spiritual convictions had a profound influence on Mr. Waterman and are reflected in many of the spiritual insights found in this book.

To my wife, Pegi
for
her compassionate insights
and loving support.

Contents

Foreword

Many counselors are able to help those in distress cope with troubling circumstances, but only the work of the Holy Spirit can bring you the peace that surpasses all understanding. On that fateful night before Jesus was crucified, there was a strange and mysterious heaviness upon the disciples' hearts. So after Jesus had told them of his betrayal and coming departure, he gave them these words of comfort, "Peace I leave with you, My peace I give to you; not as the world gives do I give to you. Let not your heart be troubled, neither let it be afraid" (John 14:27, NKJV). What did he leave for them? The Holy Spirit...the Comforter. For the Holy Spirit would apply into their lives all that Jesus accomplished through his death, burial, and resurrection: victory!

Sid Waterman is a man who has helped guide many people as they discover the peace of God. Not just by years of experience as a counselor, but through his own relationship with Jesus, the Prince of Peace. You will be touched by the testimonies of God's provision, as well as the timeless truth that comes from God's Word. For all who are struggling with the pain of loss, you will find your way to recovery as you meditate upon the insights found in this little book.

Dr. Melvin Blackaby, Ph.D.

Preface

I discovered that most books and articles I read about grief and loss do not include the mighty and compassionate work of the Holy Spirit. Yet He, the Holy Spirit, is called the Comforter—the One who comes alongside to help and heal. His gracious and supernatural power is available to those who come to Him in humble faith. He is the One who has the power and the resources to bring comfort, healing, and hope to broken, grieving hearts.

As a result, for a number of years, I have wanted to write a personal compassionate book on recovering from loss that is not only people centered but also God centered. This book combines some of the best teaching today on grief and loss with the solid biblical work of the Holy Spirit.

It can speak to anyone who is grieving. It is suitable for pastors of all denominations to give to parishioners who have suffered loss and are seeking practical and spiritual help in their journey through grief. It is easy to read and understand and is suited to people who are grieving—who are in no condition emotionally to read full-length, detailed books about grief and recovery from loss.

Acknowledgments

I wish to express my gratitude to Leanne Fairholm and Judy MacKenzie for their selfless help and encouragement in the preparation of this book.

I also must thank Tom Horn and all the staff at Anomalos Publishing. Their personal help and gracious support has been an enormous encouragement to me.

Introduction

This book, with its compassionate and personal approach, presents many practical teachings on grief and recovery from loss. Teachings, however, are not enough. We need the comfort and strength of God Himself to sustain us as we pass through the dark valley of grief and pain. When our emotions engulf us, and dark clouds cover us, we need the gracious work of the Holy Spirit to come and touch our spirits with His assurance and peace. "Is it possible" we may ask, "to have any real peace when we are filled with uneasiness and fear?" Even as we ask the question, Jesus is waiting for you to come. He longs for you to hear his strong and gentle voice:

Come to me if you are weary and tired
Come and I will give you rest
Come and cast yourself on me

Trust me and I will hold you fast
Come, just as you are with all your pain
My peace is waiting for you
Come and you will find
"I am God who is faithful and true."

1 Thessalonians 5:24, nkjv
(author's paraphrase)

This book, with its insights and practical illustrations, will help you in your journey through grief. It is also my prayer that this book will be an instrument in the hands of the Holy Spirit to bring new hope and healing as you reach out to Him.

Recovering from Loss

1

Finding God's Peace

I will never forget the day when I received a phone call from my father, who was very special to me, a man whom I loved deeply. He told me he needed me and asked me to come. He was in a hospital about five-hundred miles away. When I went to his bedside, he asked me, with great feeling, to take him home. He was very ill and wanted to spend his last days at home. After talking with his doctor, we made arrangements to take him home. I remember the contentment on his face when we tucked him into his own bed. The next day at about two o'clock in the afternoon, I felt led to join my mother in the next room and pray. I remember thanking God for my father. I thanked God for his examples of faithfulness; as a servant of God, for more than fifty years. I then prayed this prayer, "Dear Father, I sincerely ask you in Jesus' name to take Dad home to be with you. I thank you Father for hearing this prayer, in Jesus' holy name, amen." At that moment, my father stopped breathing. My mother and I rushed to his bedside. We both cried and prayed at the same time as we bid him farewell. My heart overflowed with an incredible feeling of emptiness and loss. The one I admired and loved was no longer with us. I remembered my father telling me that the greatest discovery he would ever make would be one second after he died. Although I knew he was safe in the arms of Jesus, I continued to weep and grieve.

When we experience a deep loss, our minds can be flooded with confusing and clouded thoughts. It seems our emotions are at a breaking point. Nothing seems real. The pain and grief are too much to comprehend. Sometimes reality and memories are just a big blur. There is an emptiness mixed with fear:

* fear of the future
* fear of the unknown
* fear of being alone

The one I loved deeply, who was part of my life, was gone. My ordered world had been turned upside down. I felt so helpless to do anything about it. My grief swept over me like giant waves of sorrow crashing all around me.

Sometimes one can be so overwhelmed with grief, they are beside themselves with the magnitude of the loss. I remember a lady who came to me for counseling. She had lost her twenty-four-year-old daughter. She and her daughter had been very close. In a lovely Mother's Day card, she told her mother that she was her very best friend. She thanked her mother for bringing her into the world. The love she expressed in that card to her mother moved me to tears. It reminded me of the love relation-ship between Ruth and Naomi, found in the Book of Ruth in the Old Testament.

Later, the daughter attended a concert with her boyfriend in another city. A disagreement arose and the boy left. Some friends invited her to stay the night with them in a motor home. That night the motor home caught fire. Everyone escaped except her daughter. She was missed by the rescuers in the confusion and panic of the moment. To make matters worse, the girl was to be maid-of-honor at her mother's wedding in a few weeks. The mother was so overwhelmed with grief that she could hardly breathe. It seemed she was being consumed with an indescribable inner pain. There was an empty void deep inside that had no bottom. She was beside herself. She didn't know what to do or where to go. She had read books on grieving but nothing seemed to help. She had come to the end of herself. I shared with her how God's grace was sufficient for every need we have and how His strength is made perfect in our weakness. I told her that God's grace was not only sufficient but also available to her. As she listened through her tears, it became clear that God was the only one who could fill her empty heart and bring peace. I explained to her that when Jesus' disciples were overwhelmed with fear and anxiety, He said to them, "My peace I leave with you. My peace I give to you. Do not let your hearts be troubled and don't be afraid" (John 14:27, NKJV; author's paraphrase).

I told her God's peace was beyond reason or understanding. God can bring peace when it seems peace is impossible. We say, "How can I have peace at a time like this? It doesn't make sense." I shared how God's peace is a supernatural peace. It is the peace Jesus had when He went to the cross and it is available today. It became very clear to me, as I listened and shared with her, the only thing this grieving lady could do was cast herself, with all her emptiness and grief, totally and completely upon the Lord. I asked her to let go of her crushing burden and abandon herself to Jesus. I assured her that Jesus promised to do the following:

- receive her
- comfort her
- give her rest

He said, "Come to me, yes, come to me if you are weary, tired, and burdened. I will give you rest" (Matthew 11:28, NKJV; author's paraphrase). That dear grieving lady, whose heart was so broken with grief, responded to God's gracious invitation. She prayed with me. She trusted Jesus with her past, her present, and her future. She cast all her burdens, emptiness, and pain on

Jesus. She asked the Holy Spirit to come into her life and fill her with the presence of Jesus. We prayed for the comforter to come and fill her with God's peace that passes all understanding. I remember praying for God, through His gracious Spirit, to fill her with the healing and comfort of Jesus. I prayed, "Come Holy Spirit, come with all the grace and power of Jesus and do what only you can do. I ask you in Jesus holy name to fill this lady with the amazing love of Jesus."

The Lord heard her cry for help. He came that day and touched her with His peace. He began a new work of healing in her life. With the help of the Holy Spirit, she began to walk hand-in-hand with Jesus, her Comforter, her Lord, and her Savior. However, in spite of trusting Jesus with all her pain and loss, at times, a terrible sense of grief and emptiness would return. It would overwhelm her with sorrow.

Then one day, about three weeks later, a great release came into her life. She said, "I don't know what has happened, but for the first time I feel free." A new calm and rest overshadowed her. Her countenance changed. She began to smile. A new radiance shone from her face. The Lord had heard her cry for help. He was working in her life, faithful to her even when the heavy clouds of sorrow and grief rolled in. It is most important to know that our Heavenly Father always keeps His word. You can trust Him to keep His promises. He cannot deny Himself. When the dark clouds come, remember, He is still holding your hand. Don't let go! He will lead you and carry you through the dark and discouraging times that come. This gracious lady still grieves the loss of her lovely daughter, for grief is the price we pay for love. However, she does not grieve with a spirit of hopeless despair. Yes, we grieve, but we do not grieve like those who have no hope. In the midst of our grief, we experience God's strength and peace. If we trust Him and take His hand, He will protect us and strengthen us, leading us into green pastures and beside still waters. We will know that He is with us and His strong arms will hold us fast.

2

Grief is the Price We Pay for Love

It is good to know that grief is the inevitable consequence of love. When we love someone, we enter into a love relationship—a relationship that is difficult to describe. We know there are deep emotional feelings of caring and giving that bring joy. These feelings tie us to that person in "bonds of love." We open ourselves to personal feelings of joy and fulfillment when we love someone. We also open ourselves to grief when that one is taken away. The deeper we love—the greater we grieve. It doesn't really matter how young or old he or she may be. When a love relationship is broken, we grieve.

Where there is no love
There is no grief

Where there is little love
There is little grief
Where there is much love
There is much grief

Grief, therefore, is a good thing. It is not a sign of weakness. It does not mean we are falling apart. It is a sign of deep love. It is healthy and good—good for us to express the grief that has its roots in love. When we express our grief, let us remember that God is listening to our deepest cries and our unspoken sighs. He not only listens to our hearts cry, He comes through His spirit and grieves with us.

He is the one who said, "Weep with those who weep" (Romans 12:15, NKJV). God not only weeps with us, He comes alongside and helps bear our burdens and carry our sorrows. He often does this through those who are closest to us. The Holy Spirit can use loved ones and close friends to come alongside us with the love and compassion of Jesus. This brings comfort and strength when we are overwhelmed with sorrow and loss.

Sometimes, the only way we can express our grief is with tears. I remember visiting a dear man I knew who lost his wife to a heart attack while he was away. When he returned home and discovered her, he was overwhelmed with grief. Later, while visiting him, I asked him to share with me the emotions and feelings that were inside. He put his head on my shoulder and cried and cried and cried! The tears that fell that day were more eloquent than any words in expressing the depth of loss and grief he felt. Let us not be afraid to grieve. Jesus wept. He also weeps with those who weep. Remember, He is by our side when we grieve. It is comforting to know that at times like this, we feel His spirit grieving with us. We discover the following results:

- our burdens are lighter
- our pain is softened
- we feel comforted

3

There is No Right or Wrong Way to Grieve

It is important to understand that the way we express our sorrow and grief is different for everyone. Some grieve with many tears and much emotion. Others, because of their background, personality, or culture, grieve with little emotion and few tears. There is no right or wrong way to grieve. One size does not fit all. The way we grieve is not necessarily an indication of the depth of sorrow we feel.

What relief!

What freedom!

No matter how we grieve, it is real and good. This awareness frees us from any concern about the "appropriate" way to grieve. It frees us from any comparison or judgment as to how others grieve. It also sets us free.

Grieve freely, knowing that no matter how we grieve, God understands and is by our side to help us.

The truth is, we all grieve when we suffer a deep loss. To cover it up, to pretend all is well when it is not, to deny it, or look for a panacea only makes matters worse.

Our pattern for grieving may be unpredictable. There may be times when we feel we are on the road to recovery. We are doing quite well. Then suddenly, without warning, we find ourselves overwhelmed with sorrow. The tears flow, it seems, for no apparent reason. We don't understand what is happening. This is normal. Even as our feelings for love cannot be programmed, so too, our feelings of grief for someone we love cannot be programmed.

4

Dealing with Doubt, Fear, and Guilt

At first there may be disbelief. We know the loss has occurred, but everything in our emotions cries out:

- It can't be true!
- I don't believe it!

The result may be tension between conflicting emotions. This is sometimes followed by anger. "It's not fair," we say. "Why did it happen?" "Why this way?" "Why me?" If, in the midst of grief and unanswered questions, you feel abandoned by God, or you are tempted to doubt His love for you, don't turn away from Him. Instead, trust Him with all your fears and doubts. Trust Him fully. He will come to you with His compassion and grace. He will renew you deep within. When you sense His gracious presence, His peace will come to you in spite of all the confusion and unanswered questions. Let His grace strengthen you (2 Corinthians 12:9, NKJV; author's paraphrase).

Let His arms of love surround you.

ISAIAH 40:11, NKJV

(AUTHOR'S PARAPHRASE)

Let His spirit fill you with His peace.

EPHESIANS 5:22, NKJV

(AUTHOR'S PARAPHRASE)

However, in spite of knowing His love for you, a sense of guilt can creep in and compound the burden of grief we feel. We say, "If only—if only I were there when they died."

If only I had spent more time with them
If only I had told them how much I loved them

If only we had taken that holiday we planned
  together
If only! If only! If only!

I vividly remember visiting a lady who all her life,
except for about one and a half years, had lived close to
her mother whom she loved deeply. Her mother was a
quiet, gracious, giving, thoughtful and caring lady. The
bonds of love were healthy, real, and deep. When her
mother became ill, she cared for her in her home. When
her mother had to go to the hospital, she visited her constantly and showered her with love and care. One
evening when she planned to visit her mother, she was
just too tired. That night her mother passed away. The
guilt she felt almost immobilized her.

I asked her if her mother knew how much she
loved her. She replied, "Oh yes, mother knew." I told
her the love she lavished on her mother throughout her
lifetime was accumulative. (Even as bitterness and
anger can also accumulate over time.) This love was an
integral part of her mother's life. Even though she was
not at her mother's bedside when she died—her love

was there and her mother knew it. I reassured her that her mother, who was always thinking of others rather than herself, was not resentful when she passed through the valley. The love she had "invested" in her mother over the years bore fruit in her mother's life at her time of death. As we continued to talk and pray together, her burden of guilt lifted. It was such a joy for me to see this gracious woman set free from the terrible weight of guilt that was crushing her. When I left she was still at the window waving good-bye and expressing her gratitude for what God had done in her life.

This deep desire in our hearts, wishing we had done more, is always an expression of love. This is the nature of love and it is good. Let this awareness comfort you. Remember, the one you lost

* knew your heart of love,
* experienced your care and concern,
* and was the recipient of your love.

Do not allow guilt to come, accuse you, and lay burdens on you. The enemy of our souls always comes and accuses us in times of weakness. It is Jesus who comes and lifts our burdens and removes our guilt. Sometimes He is the only one who can do it. If you ask Him, He will.

However, there are times when the burden of guilt is so great we find it almost impossible to forgive ourselves. I will never forget a young lady in her early thirties who came to me with a crushing burden of guilt. She was helpless to do anything about it. Her only option, she felt, was to run away and move across the country. The story she told me will be forever etched in my mind. The young man she had married was too good to be true. His deep and strong character was permeated with amazing love and thoughtfulness. He loved his wife with all his heart. She was God's special gift wrapped in love. Although she deeply loved and cherished him, at times her vibrant temperament would come out. One morning as he was leaving for work they had a disagreement. On this occasion, the disagreement grew into a conflict. As he walked out the door she told him to "Get out." As soon as he left she felt terrible. At about three o'clock there was a knock at the door. When she opened the door, the deliveryman handed her a dozen roses with a card. She opened the card and read,

"To my dear wife. I am so sorry for what happened this morning. I love you with all my heart." It was signed, "Your loving husband." She was reminded again of the amazing husband God had given her. At about five o'clock, there was another knock at the door. This time it was a police officer. There had been a terrible head-on collision on the highway and her husband had been instantly killed. The last words she had said to her husband were "Get Out." And the last words he said to her, graced with a dozen roses, were, "I love you with all my heart." This young lady's guilt and grief was overwhelming. It was like a tsunami. She was inundated, swept away, tossed to and fro. She could never forgive herself. I have counseled those who believe that God in His great mercy can and will forgive them. They also know, like this young lady, that the one they had hurt would forgive them. However, they find it impossible to ever forgive themselves. They find themselves locked into a prison of guilt and hopelessness.

If you, for whatever reason, find it impossible to forgive yourself, I have good news for you.

If God has heard your prayer and forgiven you,

who are you not to forgive yourself? Are you more righteous than God? Do you have higher standards than God? Are you holier than God? Are you bigger than God? If you are forgiven by God, you are fully, completely, and totally forgiven. God's forgiveness, like everything else He does, is perfect. When you accept His perfect and complete forgiveness you know you are fully forgiven. The Holy Spirit will come and confirm this in your heart and give you the grace to forgive yourself. To be truly forgiven by a Holy God is to be set free. Pray this prayer and the truth will set you free.

My Dear Father in Heaven,
I praise you for your amazing love for me.
I praise you for your mercy that endures forever.
I praise you for your forgiveness through Jesus.
I praise you that you cleanse me from all
guilt through the blood of Jesus.
I repent of my sin of unbelief.
I turn from my sin and doubt.

I reach out and accept your amazing forgiveness.
Thank you Lord, I am forgiven. You have set me free.
I love you. You are my Lord and my God.
I pray this prayer with thanksgiving in my
heart to you my dear, dear Heavenly Father.
In Jesus' name, Amen.

LUKE 11:2, NKJV

(AUTHOR'S PARAPHRASE)

If you sincerely prayed this prayer you are free—free to forgive yourself. Your burden of guilt is gone. There are no more clouds hanging over you. As far as you can see, your horizons are clear. God is pleased with you. You are His child. All is well. May the reality of this amazing truth flood your soul with God's peace as you continue your journey of recovering from your loss.

5

God Has a Purpose
for Your Life

It is possible to allow the pain and enormity of the loss to overwhelm you. You feel too helpless to do anything about it and you may be tempted to give up. Your hopes have been shattered. Your dreams have evaporated. You say to yourself, "What's the use?"

Over the years, people have said to me, "What can you do? The one I loved is gone—gone forever. Nothing will be the same again. You can't do anything to change what has happened." It is true that nothing will be the same again. It can't be. The one you loved and was a part of your life is gone. This, however, does not mean that your life cannot be good again. Although, your life will be different, and change is never easy, it is important to believe that your life can have purpose and meaning again. God will reveal His purpose for you as you ask Him and follow His leading. Psalm 139 makes it abundantly clear that God formed you and knit you together in your mother's womb. Nothing was hidden from Him. All your days on earth were planned and ordained for you before one of them came to be. In fact, the psalmist tells us that they were all written in your book before you were born. This includes what God has planned for you today, tomorrow, and for the rest of your life.

6

Your Response Is Your Key to Recovery

The way you respond to the loss in your life will determine the joy and quality of life you can experience in the future. When my wife and I lived in Kentucky, we were told we must go to hear a brilliant young man who was establishing a reputation as an outstanding speaker.

The Sunday we went to hear him, he told us about the death of his ten-year-old daughter. He told us about the time when it became obvious that something was seriously wrong. Tests revealed she had a severe strain of leukemia. The prognosis was not good. Slowly she began to fail. The fear and pain they felt as they saw their beautiful little daughter grow weaker and weaker was beyond words. One day she looked at her father and asked, "Daddy, am I going to die?"

What do you say to your little girl in reply to such a personal and heart-wrenching question? The day came when she died. He told us that his initial response was one of bitterness and anger. It is one thing when a rose comes to full bloom and its petals slowly fall away, losing all of its beauty. It is quite another when a bursting bud is blasted by a killing frost. As he began to walk down the path of anger and bitterness, he discovered it began to infect his whole life. Everything he did, even the way he conducted himself and how he spoke, seemed to reflect this inner turmoil. He realized that he was slowly becoming a bitter man. He recognized that this path led nowhere. He then chose to walk down another path. He called it the path of silent resignation. Life did not make sense. He resigned himself to a kind of fatalistic "whatever will be, will be." As he walked down this path, he told us that life began to lose all meaning and purpose. It began to affect not only his own outlook on life, but it also affected others around him. He recognized that this path of silent resignation was not good. As he contemplated all this, he remembered an incident when he was a little boy. His family was poor. They had no washing machine. One day family friends, who were going overseas to help in the war effort, decided to lend their washing machine to his mother while they were away. Every Saturday, he would go downstairs and help his mother wash. It was exciting and fun to watch the agitator churn back and forth, filling the machine with suds. One day, about two-and-a-half years later, he went downstairs and two men were carrying the machine out the door.

He ran upstairs and cried out to his mother, "Mommy, mommy, they're taking away our washing machine!" His mother put an arm around him and said, "My dear son, this washing machine was never ours in the first place. It was given to us for a time—to be a help and a blessing. The family that owned it is taking it back. Our only response is one of thanksgiving and gratitude for the two-and-a-half years we had it." As he related this story to the death of his daughter, he began to give thanks to the Lord for the ten precious years they had together. He realized that if he had the choice never to have had his daughter, and therefore, never to have to experience the pain, grief, and agony of watching her slowly pass away, or to have her for only ten years and go through the terrible sense of emptiness and loss when she died, there would be no choice. The love and joy she brought to the home was greater than the pain and sorrow of losing her. As he began to walk down this third path, he found himself giving thanks for everything:

- for each new day
- for the blue sky and clouds
- for family and friends
- for the gift of life itself

This spirit of thanksgiving began to infect his whole life. It is true. Something happens when we put our hand in the hand of God and begin to thank Him for His love and faithfulness. We discover this spirit of thanksgiving is a healing spirit that brings new freedom and joy. The future that seemed so dark begins to change. Rays of hope come and our life begins to be filled with new purpose and meaning. It affects who we are and what we do. Trusting our Heavenly Father and giving thanks to Him is therapy to a grieving heart. As we remember and thank Him for the good times and the precious memories, our empty hearts are not quite so empty. It is good to take a piece of paper and write down all the things in the past for which you are truly thankful. Use this list as a guide for your prayer time. Find a close friend or loved one to share it with. It will be difficult but it will be good. The path you walk down is a choice.

You can trust the Lord and thank Him for His goodness to you over the years in good times and bad, or you can allow the loss of the one you love hold you fast and determine your future. This will result in a sense of helplessness. This can lead to doubt, discouragement, and even despair. However, you also can choose to believe that God is with you and, in His wisdom and grace, has a purpose for you. His plan for you is not finished. He wants you to enjoy Him, love life, serve Him, and be an encouragement to others. Seek His leading. Take His hand. Let Him lead you into green pastures and beside still waters. He will restore your soul.

HEALING A BROKEN HEART

My response to the loss
Of the one I loved
Can help or hinder
My journey through grief.

I can choose to give thanks
For the life we shared
As together in love
Through good times and bad
We laughed and we cared.

When we hold on to hurts
Or give in to despair
It can rob us of hope
The future looks dark
I really don't care.

It is true, my new life
Will not be the same
It can't be, the one I love
Is no longer with me.

Although change is hard
And my grief is deep
God has a purpose
For me to keep.
God's purpose and plan are the very best
Take His hand and follow Him
He will give you,
His peace and rest.

He will lead you in green pastures
He will satisfy your soul
His strength will come and lift you up
And when you come just as you are
And give your broken heart to Him
He will make you whole.

Put your hand in the hand of God. It will be better
than a light and safer than knowing the way. Apply this
powerful principle everyday as you continue your journey through grief. There are times in life when you
have no control of: What people say or do to you, what
happens to you, or the circumstances you are in. The

only thing you have control over is your response to what is happening. You have a choice. You can respond in the spirit of God as Jesus did, when He said, "Father, forgive them they don't know what they are doing" (Luke 23:34, NKJV; author's paraphrase), or you can respond emotionally. Your response determines your peace of mind. It is so easy to respond in a spirit of hurt or anger. This leads to conflict both inside and out. The result is frustration and damaged or even broke relationships. If, however, through God's grace and the power of the Holy Spirit, you respond like Jesus, healing and reconciliation can take place. Remember, the greatest and most important thing in your life is not your circumstances or what happens to you. It is your response. When hurtful or painful things happen to you, pause to pray, seek God's face, cry out to the one who said, "Ask and you will receive, seek and you will find" (Luke 11:9, NKJV). This is the abundant life Jesus promises. It is a life under God's control. Believe that "God is able to do exceedingly, abundantly more than we could ever imagine" (Ephesians 3:20, NKJV; author's paraphrase), and you will be set free. Free to forgive.

Free to love, even the unlovely. Free to live in the freedom and joy that Jesus gives. What a way to live! It is God's way. It is the only way. It is the way of healing and hope. Your recovery from hurt and loss is determined by your response empowered and lead by the Holy Spirit.

Turn and face the sunrise each new day, giving thanks for His love and His leading. You will discover a new joy in living and new purpose and direction in life. Events and circumstances will no longer dictate your joy or your future—God will. Your life will become a new adventure as you walk hand-in-hand with Him.

7

Unresolved Issues

What do we do if there were issues or problems with the one we lost that were never dealt with before he or she died? For whatever reason, we did not reconcile, forgive, ask forgiveness, or make things right before the death. These unresolved issues may include the following:

* words that were spoken or unspoken
* attitudes that were expressed or not expressed
* decisions that, in retrospect, were not good

These can linger like a dark cloud hanging over your head. We ask ourselves the question, "What can I do?" Then we answer our own question by saying, "It's too late to do anything, they are no longer here." The result may be a sense of helplessness, guilt, discouragement, or even anger. If you are in this difficult situation, the good news is, there is something you can do. It can be very helpful and healing to sit down and write a personal letter to the one you have lost. This letter is not for the benefit of the one you loved. You are writing this letter for your own healing and recovery. When you write your letter, address your loved one by name. Begin by telling the one you lost how much you loved them. It is important to be specific, personal, and real. If you need to say you are sorry and ask for forgiveness, or if you need to forgive them for something they have done to you, be specific. Remember when you forgive others you release God's forgiveness in your life. When you forgive, you open the door to God's forgiveness. This sets you free from the guilt and bondage of an unforgiving spirit. Conclude your letter by thanking them for their love and the good times you had together. When you say goodbye, remember you are not saying goodbye to your love for them, or their love for you. You are not saying goodbye to the good times you had together. You are not saying goodbye to precious memories. You are saying goodbye to the physical relationship that will never be again. It is most important that you find a trusted friend or loved one—one who cares and understands. Share with your friend what you have done. Pray together, and then read your letter. This will be one of the most profound and difficult things you have ever done. When you do this you will experience God's presence and a new release deep inside. You will discover the following:

- your burdens are not quite so heavy
- your future will look brighter
- the next chapter in your life will come into clearer focus
- life will become full and free

8

Uncertainty about Eternity

A great burden that can hinder your recovery is the uncertainty you have regarding your loved one's relationship with Jesus before they died. You may be concerned because they never prayed the prayer that you feel is necessary for them to truly know God and His forgiveness. The clear teaching from scripture is that God, through His spirit, is constantly seeking us. In the story of the lost sheep (Luke 15:3–7, NKJV), the shepherd went out into the hills searching, looking and seeking until it was found. It does not say he looked until he was tired or exhausted and returned home. The shepherd didn't say, "I will teach that stubborn, willful sheep a lesson and let him go." No, he continued looking until it was found, in spite of pain and hardship. This is the same shepherd who, through the Holy

Spirit, was reaching out and pursuing your loved one before he or she died. We are told in scripture that "whosoever will call on the name of the Lord will be saved" (Romans 10:13, NKJV; author's paraphrase). When the spirit comes and reveals Jesus, His love and forgiveness, who He is and what He has done, deep in the soul, all one has to do is say, "My Lord and my God." You can rest assured that one is safe in the arms of Jesus. It is comforting to know that although we see only the "outside," God looks at the heart. God heard every one of your prayers. He came by His spirit and reached out in love and grace to your loved one. He stood by their side listening for the faintest cry of their soul, longing to forgive and ready to accept. "God is not willing that any should perish but for everyone to come to repentance" (2 Peter 3:9, NKJV; author's paraphrase). In response, we cry out with the hymn writer:

> Jesus, what a friend for sinners
> Jesus, lover of my soul
> Jesus, what a help in sorrow
> While the billows o'er me roll

Hallelujah! What a Saviour
Hallelujah! What a friend
Saving, helping, keeping, loving
He is with me to the end.

> (Taken from the hymn "Our Great Saviour,"
> verses 1 and 3, and chorus. J. Wilbur Chapman,
> *New Church Hymnal* (Lexicon Music Incorporated,
> International copyright 1976), 23.)

May this amazing truth of His amazing love comfort you with his assurance and peace.

9

Finding God's Healing and Power through Prayer

In many ways, life is like a book. The opening chapter began with your birth. Growing up as a child was a chapter filled with wonderment and adventure. Then came the time to leave home. In this chapter, you faced new challenges and made new friends. Many more chapters followed. Everyone's book is unique and different. For some, their book includes getting married, having a family, and finally retiring. For others, their book does not follow the "normal" script. Each book has its own twists and turns, with its joys and sorrows. The sorrow and loss you have just experienced has interrupted your latest chapter. Because of the nature and depth of the loss you may feel that no more good chapters can be written. Let me assure you, with God at your side and the Holy Spirit leading you and giving you strength, the next chapter in your life can be filled with the adventure of walking with God, discovering His goodness and looking forward with anticipation to what God has in store for you. The key is to trust the One who said, "I will never leave you nor forsake you." Thank Him for His love and compassion:

I thank you Lord
For your caring heart
For a person such as me
The fact, that you almighty God
With all your power and might
Reach out in love to me
Eases my pain and comforts me
In my sorrow and my night

I thank you God you love me so
So very much indeed!
Your tender heart
Your love and grace

Meets my every need
Help me O Lord
To love and care
For those who have suffered loss
That they may know
Your heart of love
That gives at any cost
Your amazing grace
Is beyond compare
You gave your life for me
You come and fill my life with peace
Your grace has set me free

I love you Lord
I really do!
I give my life afresh
For you to come, and fill me now
With your perfect peace and rest.

As you pray this prayer, you will discover the healing grace of God flooding through your soul. With the
love and grace you have received, reach out, and comfort

others in their time of loss. Take your "five loaves and two fish" and ask God to bless them and use them to bless those around you. When you see God answering your prayers through the love you have given to others, you will come alive with the love of Jesus. You will find a new joy in your life as you see God's power flowing through you to help and encourage others. "Now, may the God of peace equip you for doing His will and may He work in you what is pleasing to Him, to Him be glory forever and ever, Amen" (Hebrews 13:20, 21, NJKV; author's paraphrase).

A Prayer for Those Who Are Grieving

Lord, I come to you and I don't know what to say. I am so full of emptiness and fear. I have so many questions. My mind is confused and my emotions are so deep. I hurt so much. I think my heart is going to break. I feel so helpless to do anything about the situation. It seems nothing can be done. My loss is so final. Lord, what can I do? I come to you, Oh Lord. I know you understand better than anyone else. You suffered more than I will ever know. In the garden you cried out in terrible agony. You wept—your tears and sweat were like drops of blood falling to the ground. Your soul was wrung out to the very point of death. On the cross you cried out, "My God, my God, why have you forsaken me?"

(Matthew 27:46, NJKV). Lord, I will never know how "deep were the waters crossed, or how dark the night you went through" (Elizabeth Clephane, "There Were Ninety and Nine," *Sankey's Songs and Solos* (Harper Collins 2005)). I believe it was for me, to bring me forgiveness and hope, healing and help in my time of need. So Lord, I come to you. I thank you for your sufferings for

* It is by your wounds that I am healed.
* It is through your love that I am lifted up.
* It is through your resurrection I have hope.
* It is through the Holy Spirit—the comforter, I find comfort.
* It is through your presence I find peace.
* It is through your death, I find life.

I thank you that your word tells me:

Do not fear
I have called you by name
You are mine

When you pass through the waters I am with you
When you pass through the rivers
They will not sweep over you.

When you walk through the fire
You will not be burned
The flames will not set you ablaze
For I am the Lord
And I am your God
I am the Holy One of Israel
And I am your Saviour.

ISAIAH 43:1–2, NIV

(AUTHOR'S PARAPHRASE)

Lord, I come to you today. I come with all my burdens, fears, and doubts. I cast myself on you. I trust you with all I am and all I have. I give myself completely to you. I ask you to comfort me with your love. Fill me with your peace. Help me to trust you knowing that you are hearing and answering this prayer. You are my Lord and my God.

I thank you Lord for your peace that fills my soul. I

thank you for your healing and comfort through your gracious spirit. I thank you for your faithfulness to me. Lord, I know I am not alone—you are with me—forever.

I praise you, that you will carry me through the darkness and doubt of my soul. How I praise you! You have everything under control. You said, "I will never leave you nor forsake you" (Hebrews 13:5, NKJV). How I love you! You are my Father, my Lord, my comfort, my peace and my hope.

Lord, thank you for inviting me to come. You said, "Come to me if you are weary and burdened down with care, I will give you rest" (Matthew 11:28, NKJV; author's paraphrase). Lord, you also said, "My peace I leave with you. My peace I give to you...Let not your heart be troubled, neither let it be afraid" (John 14:27, KJV).

Thank you Lord for your gracious Holy Spirit who fills me with the peace of Jesus. I love you Lord. You are my rock and my salvation, whom shall I fear.

Lord,

You are my anchor ~ In the storm
You are my light ~ In darkness

You are my comfort~In sorrow

You are my hope~In despair

You are my peace~In troubled waters

You are my strength~In weakness

You are my life~In death

I praise you, that through Jesus you are my Father;

You love me,

You are with me,

Your strong arms are around me,

You will never leave me nor forsake me,

HEBREWS 13:5, NKJV

(AUTHOR'S PARAPHRASE)

Your grace is sufficient for me,

2 CORINTHIANS 12:9, NKJV

(AUTHOR'S PARAPHRASE)

Your strength and power are available to me.

I pray this in the name of the Father, the Son, and the gracious Holy Spirit. Amen.

Bibliography

John W. James and Russel Friedman, *The Grief Recovery Handbook* (New York: Harper Perennial, 1998).

Suggested Uses for This Book

This book would be an excellent resource for pastors to give to those in their congregation who have suffered a deep loss. It could also be used by members of a congregation to give to their friends and loved ones who are bereaved. If a sample copy were sent to pastors of churches with the above suggestions, it would have great potential to minister to thousands in their time of need. Making this book available to military, prison, or hospital chaplains and to Christian recovery from addiction centers are also possibilities.

Sid Waterman